GASTRIC BARIATRIC COOKBOOK FOR BEGINNERS

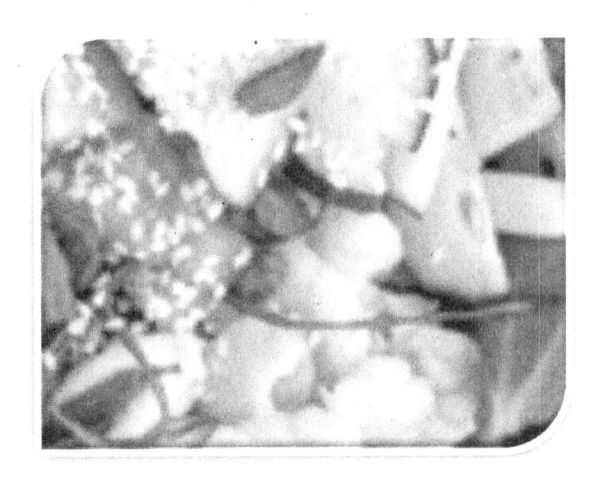

Healthy and Post-Surgery Recipes with a 30-Day Meal Plan and Nutritional Guidance for Rapid Weight Loss.

Dr. Linda B. Allen

Copyright©2024 by Dr. Linda B. Allen

All rights reserved. No part of this book may be reproduced, distributed, or transmitted in any form or by any means, including photocopying, recording, or other Electronic or mechanical methods, without the prior written permission of the author, except in the case of brief Quotations embodied in critical reviews and certain other Non-commercial uses permitted by copyright law. For Permission requests, write to the author, addressed "Attention: Permissions Coordinator,"

[dr.lindahelp@gmail.com].

EXTRA BONUS

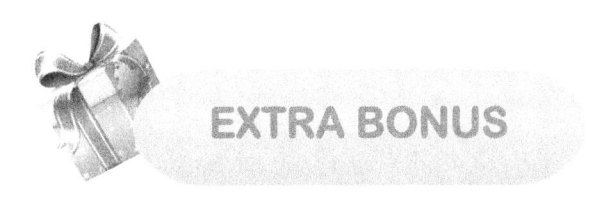

BONUS NO. 1

WEEKLY MEAL PLANNER

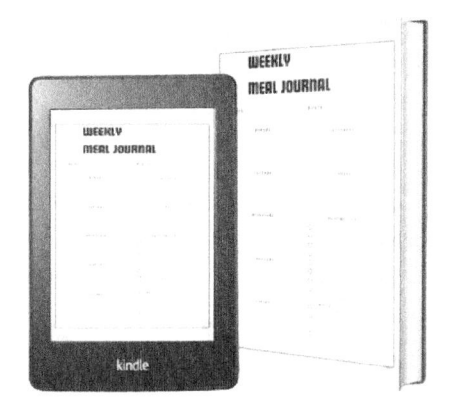

BONUS NO. 2

NUTRITIONAL GUIDANCE AND TIPS

SCAN THE QR-CODE BELOW FOR MORE BOOKS FROM THIS AUTHOR

TABLE OF CONTENTS

INTRODUCTION 9
   Overview of Gastric Sleeve Surgery 10
   Importance of Nutrition Post-Surgery 11
   How This Cookbook Can Help 12

UNDERSTANDING THE GASTRIC SLEEVE SURGERY ... 15
   What is Gastric Sleeve Surgery? 15
   What Happens During Gastric Sleeve Surgery? 16
   How Does Vertical Sleeve Gastrectomy Differ from a Bypass Surgery Procedure? 17
   What Are the Benefits of a Sleeve Gastrectomy? 18
   What Are the Risks Associated with the Procedure? 20

UNDERSTANDING THE GASTRIC SLEEVE DIET 23
   Preparing for Surgery: Dietary Guidelines 23
   Post-Surgery Dietary Phases 25
   Nutritional Requirements for Gastric Sleeve Patients 27

ESSENTIAL KITCHEN TOOLS AND INGREDIENTS 31
   Must-Have Kitchen Equipment 31
   Stocking Your Pantry with Healthy Ingredients 33
   Shopping Tips for Bariatric-Friendly Foods 36

NUTRITIONAL GUIDANCE AND TIPS 39
   Portion Control and Mindful Eating 39
   Tips for Portion Control 40
   Meeting Micronutrient Needs 40
   Key Micronutrients to Focus On 41

DELICIOUS AND POST-SURGERY RECIPES 43

BREAKFAST RECIPES 43
1. Berry Blast Protein Smoothie 43
2. Apple Cinnamon Protein Oatmeal 44
3. Spinach and Feta Egg Muffins 45
4. Chia Seed Pudding Parfait 46
5. Cottage Cheese and Pineapple Protein Bowl 47
6. Avocado and Turkey Breakfast Wrap 48
7. Blueberry Protein Pancakes 49
8. Greek Yogurt Parfait with Almond Granola 50
9. Quinoa Breakfast Bowl 51
10. Savory Veggie and Cheese Omelette 52

LUNCH RECIPES 53
1. Grilled Chicken Salad with Balsamic Vinaigrette 53
2. Quinoa and Black Bean Bowl 54
3. Salmon and Vegetable Stir-Fry 55
4. Turkey and Veggie Lettuce Wraps 56
5. Vegetarian Quiche Cups 57
6. Mediterranean Chickpea Salad 58
7. Egg Salad Lettuce Wraps 59
8. Shrimp and Avocado Zoodle Bowl 60
9. Stuffed Bell Peppers with Ground Chicken 61
10. Tuna and Avocado Lettuce Wraps 62

DINNER RECIPES 63
1. Baked Lemon Herb Chicken 63
2. Cauliflower Fried Rice with Shrimp 64
3. Turkey and Vegetable Skewers 65

4. Salmon and Asparagus Foil Packets 66
5. Eggplant Lasagna with Ground Chicken 67
6. Chicken and Vegetable Stir-Fry 68
7. Vegetarian Zucchini Noodles with Pesto...................... 69
8. Shredded Chicken Lettuce Wraps................................. 70
9. Cabbage and Turkey Casserole...................................... 71
10. Cilantro Lime Grilled Shrimp Salad........................... 72

SNACK RECIPES 73
1. Greek Yogurt Parfait with Berries 73
2. Cottage Cheese and Pineapple Bowl 74
3. Hard-Boiled Egg and Avocado Slices 75
4. Protein-Packed Trail Mix.. 76
5. Vegetable Sticks with Hummus.................................... 77
6. Turkey and Cheese Roll-Ups.. 78
7. Caprese Skewers with Cherry Tomatoes and Mozzarella
.... 79
8. Edamame and Sea Salt.. 80
9. Baked Kale Chips 81
10. Protein-Packed Cottage Cheese Bowl 82

DESSERT AND TREAT RECIPES 83
1. Chia Seed Pudding with Berries 83
2. Baked Apple with Cinnamon.. 84
3. Protein-Packed Chocolate Mousse 85
4. Frozen Banana Bites 86
5. Coconut and Almond Energy Balls 87
6. Yogurt and Berry Parfait... 88
7. Pumpkin Spice Protein Bites 89

8. Avocado Chocolate Mousse 90
9. Berry Sorbet.. 91
10. Almond Butter Stuffed Dates 92
BARIATRIC-FRIENDLY SOUPS AND SALADS............ 93
1. Tomato Basil Soup 93
2. Chicken and Vegetable Soup.. 94
3. Spinach and Feta Salad 95
4. Broccoli Cheddar Soup.. 96
5. Turkey and Cranberry Salad.. 97
6. Cauliflower and Leek Soup 98
7. Shrimp and Avocado Salad.. 99
8. Butternut Squash Soup... 100
9. Quinoa and Chickpea Salad....................................... 101
10. Asparagus and Mushroom Soup 102
30-DAY MEAL PLAN 103
CONCLUSION 113
WEEKLY MEAL PLANNER 115

8 | Gastric Sleeve Bariatric Cookbook for Beginners

INTRODUCTION

Embarking on a journey towards wellness is a profound and personal decision, often driven by a desire for a healthier and more fulfilling life. If you are holding this book, it means you or someone dear to you has taken that courageous step toward transformation through gastric sleeve bariatric surgery. Welcome to the "Gastric Sleeve Bariatric Cookbook for Beginners: Healthy and Post-Surgery Recipes with a 30-Day Meal Plan and Nutritional Guidance for Rapid Weight Loss." This isn't just a cookbook; it's a companion on your path to recovery, health, and vitality.

Let me share a personal story that fueled the creation of this cookbook. My cousin sister faced the challenges of gastric sleeve bariatric surgery, and witnessing her journey ignited a passion within me to provide support in a unique way. Drawing upon my love for cooking and a commitment to her well-being, I set out to create a collection of recipes specifically tailored for those navigating the post-surgery landscape.

My cousin's recovery was not only swift but remarkable. The meals I prepared, guided by the principles of nutrition crucial for post-gastric sleeve surgery, played a pivotal role in her healing. Witnessing her regaining strength, energy, and joy inspired me to extend this support to others in similar journeys.

As I shared the recipes and nutritional guidance with my cousin, something magical unfolded. The positive impact on her recovery resonated beyond the confines of our family. Friends, acquaintances, and even strangers seeking assistance in their post-bariatric surgery nutrition journey approached me. The overwhelming success stories and gratitude from those who embraced this cookbook fueled my commitment to making this resource widely available.

Overview of Gastric Sleeve Surgery:

Gastric sleeve surgery, also known as sleeve gastrectomy, involves the reduction of the stomach size to encourage weight loss. This surgical intervention restricts the amount of food the stomach can hold, leading to both physical and hormonal changes that contribute to significant and sustainable weight loss.

While the surgery itself is a powerful tool, its success is profoundly influenced by the postoperative care, especially in terms of nutrition.

Importance of Nutrition Post-Surgery:

Imagine your body as a finely tuned machine, and post-gastric sleeve surgery, it requires optimal fuel to operate at its best. Nutrition takes center stage in this transformative journey. The reduced stomach capacity necessitates a shift in dietary choices, emphasizing nutrient-dense foods to meet the body's nutritional requirements. This isn't just about weight loss; it's about nourishing your body to promote healing, sustain energy levels, and foster overall well-being.

In the initial phases post-surgery, there is a delicate balance between providing the body with essential nutrients and adjusting to the new normal. This is where the right guidance becomes paramount. The recipes and meal plan in this cookbook are meticulously crafted to align with the nutritional needs of individuals who have undergone gastric sleeve surgery. Each dish is a testament to the fusion of flavor and health, ensuring that the journey to weight loss is not only effective but also enjoyable.

How This Cookbook Can Help:

This cookbook is more than a compilation of recipes; it's a comprehensive guide crafted with care and empathy. Here's how it can be your steadfast companion on the path to recovery and wellness:

Tailored for Success: The recipes in this cookbook are thoughtfully designed to meet the unique dietary requirements post-gastric sleeve surgery. From protein-packed breakfasts to satisfying dinners, each dish is a step toward your health goals.

Nutritional Guidance: Beyond the recipes, you'll find invaluable nutritional insights and guidance. Learn about the essential nutrients your body needs, portion control, and mindful eating to make informed choices that contribute to your well-being.

30-Day Meal Plan: Take the guesswork out of meal planning with a structured 30-day meal plan. This plan ensures variety, balance, and simplicity, making it easier for you to focus on your recovery without the stress of planning each meal.

Practical Tips and Tools: Discover essential kitchen tools, ingredients, and shopping tips that will streamline your culinary journey. This cookbook is not just about what to cook but how to make the entire process seamless and enjoyable.

A Source of Inspiration: Real success stories and testimonials from individuals who have embraced these recipes and nutritional principles provide inspiration and motivation. You're not alone on this journey, and the shared experiences within these pages are a testament to the transformative power of mindful eating.

As you embark on this transformative journey, let this cookbook be your trusted guide, offering not just recipes but a roadmap to a healthier and more vibrant you. Your well-being is at the heart of every page, and I invite you to savor the flavors of health and happiness within these recipes. The journey toward rapid weight loss and sustained wellness starts here.

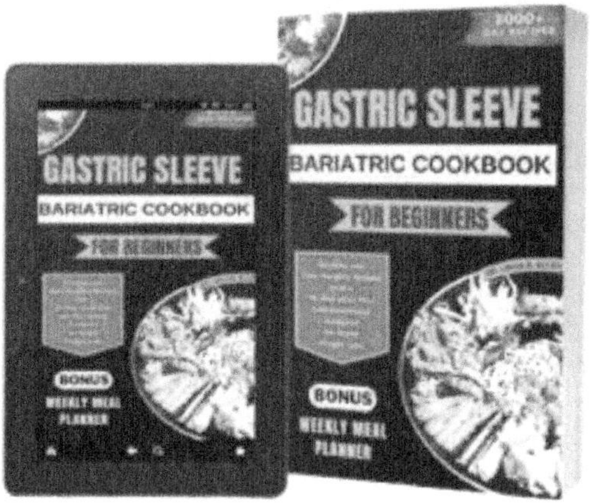
GASTRIC SLEEVE
BARIATRIC COOKBOOK
FOR BEGINNERS
BONUS
WEEKLY MEAL
PLANNER
GASTRIC SLEEVE
BARIATRIC COOKBOOK
FOR BEGINNERS
BONUS
WEEKLY MEAL
PLANNER

UNDERSTANDING THE GASTRIC SLEEVE SURGERY

Embarking on the journey towards a healthier lifestyle often involves making profound choices. For many individuals, the decision to undergo gastric sleeve surgery, also known as sleeve gastrectomy, is a transformative step towards achieving significant and sustained weight loss. In this section, we will delve into the intricacies of gastric sleeve surgery, exploring what it is, what happens during the procedure, how it differs from other weight loss surgeries, the benefits it offers, and the associated risks.

What is Gastric Sleeve Surgery?

Gastric sleeve surgery is a type of bariatric surgery that involves the removal of a large portion of the stomach, leaving behind a sleeve-shaped pouch. This procedure is designed to limit the amount of food the stomach can hold, leading to reduced calorie intake and, consequently, significant weight loss. The surgery is considered a restrictive procedure, meaning it focuses on restricting the size of the stomach to control food intake.

During the surgery, a surgeon carefully removes approximately 75-80% of the stomach, creating a smaller, banana-shaped stomach or sleeve. This smaller stomach not only reduces the amount of food that can be consumed at one time but also results in hormonal changes that contribute to decreased appetite.

What Happens During Gastric Sleeve Surgery?

The gastric sleeve surgery procedure is typically performed laparoscopically, which involves making small incisions in the abdomen through which a laparoscope (a tiny camera) and surgical instruments are inserted. This minimally invasive approach offers several advantages, including faster recovery times and reduced risk of complications.

Once the laparoscope is in place, the surgeon carefully removes a large portion of the stomach, leaving only the sleeve-shaped section. The remaining stomach is sealed using staples, creating a narrow tube or sleeve. The entire procedure takes about 1-2 hours, and most patients can expect to return home within a day or two after surgery.

How Does Vertical Sleeve Gastrectomy Differ from a Bypass Surgery Procedure?

Gastric sleeve surgery differs from gastric bypass surgery, another common bariatric procedure. While both surgeries aim to promote weight loss, they achieve this goal through different mechanisms.

In gastric sleeve surgery, the focus is on reducing the size of the stomach, limiting food intake, and altering hormonal signals related to hunger. This makes the procedure a restrictive one, as it physically restricts the amount of food the stomach can hold.

On the other hand, gastric bypass surgery combines both restrictive and malabsorptive elements. During gastric bypass, the surgeon creates a small stomach pouch and then reroutes a portion of the small intestine, causing the food to bypass the first part of the small intestine. This not only limits the amount of food the stomach can hold but also reduces the absorption of calories and nutrients.

Choosing between gastric sleeve surgery and gastric bypass depends on various factors, including individual health conditions, preferences, and the recommendations of the medical team. Both procedures have proven to be effective in promoting weight loss and improving overall health.

What Are the Benefits of a Sleeve Gastrectomy?

Gastric sleeve surgery offers a multitude of benefits beyond just weight loss. Understanding these advantages can motivate individuals to consider this procedure as a powerful tool in their journey toward better health:

Significant and Sustainable Weight Loss: The primary goal of gastric sleeve surgery is to promote substantial weight loss. Many individuals experience rapid weight loss in the first-year post-surgery, with ongoing and sustained progress.

Improved Metabolic Health: Beyond weight loss, gastric sleeve surgery often leads to improvements in metabolic conditions such as type 2 diabetes, high blood pressure, and high cholesterol. These positive changes contribute to an overall enhancement of metabolic health.

Reduced Hunger and Increased Satiety: The alteration of the stomach's size and hormonal changes post-surgery result in reduced appetite and increased feelings of fullness. This shift in hunger and satiety cues supports individuals in making healthier food choices and controlling portion sizes.

Enhanced Quality of Life: Many individuals who undergo gastric sleeve surgery report improvements in their overall quality of life. Beyond the physical benefits, the surgery often leads to increased mobility, improved self-esteem, and a greater ability to engage in various activities.

Less Invasive Procedure: The laparoscopic approach to gastric sleeve surgery minimizes scarring, reduces the risk of infection, and shortens recovery times compared to traditional open surgery.

Simplicity in Postoperative Care: Post-surgery, the maintenance and care of the sleeve-shaped stomach are relatively straightforward. The simplicity of postoperative management enhances the long-term success of the procedure.

What Are the Risks Associated with the Procedure?

While gastric sleeve surgery is generally considered safe, as with any surgical procedure, it comes with inherent risks. It is crucial for individuals considering this surgery to be aware of potential complications. However, understanding these risks should not deter one from pursuing the procedure, as the benefits often outweigh the potential drawbacks. Some common risks associated with gastric sleeve surgery include:

Infection: Infections at the incision sites or within the abdominal cavity can occur, although they are relatively rare.

Bleeding: Excessive bleeding during or after surgery is a potential risk, although this is closely monitored and managed by the surgical team.

Leakage: In some cases, the staples used to seal the remaining stomach may lead to leakage. This can result in infections or other complications and may require additional surgical intervention.

Gastroesophageal Reflux Disease (GERD): Some individuals may experience an increase in acid reflux symptoms post-surgery. This can typically be managed with lifestyle changes and, in some cases, medication.

Nutritional Deficiencies: With the reduced stomach size, there is a risk of inadequate nutrient absorption. Regular monitoring and appropriate supplementation, as advised by healthcare professionals, can mitigate this risk.

Obstruction: Rarely, the new stomach sleeve may narrow, leading to a blockage that can cause nausea, vomiting, and other symptoms. This may require further intervention.

It is essential to approach gastric sleeve surgery with a well-informed and realistic mindset. Regular follow-ups with healthcare providers, adherence to postoperative guidelines, and an understanding of potential risks contribute to a smoother and more successful recovery.

As you consider the path of gastric sleeve surgery, envision it not just as a surgical intervention but as a journey towards health and renewal.

The benefits are not solely about shedding pounds but about gaining a newfound sense of self, improved metabolic health, and the potential for a more active and fulfilling life.

In the pages of this cookbook, you will find not just recipes but a holistic approach to post-gastric sleeve surgery nutrition. The understanding of the surgery's intricacies, and expertly crafted meal plans, will guide you on your journey to rapid weight loss and sustained wellness. Let this be the beginning of a chapter in your life where health takes center stage, and the transformative power of gastric sleeve surgery becomes a catalyst for a vibrant and thriving you.

UNDERSTANDING THE GASTRIC SLEEVE DIET

The gastric sleeve diet is a critical component of post-surgery care, playing a vital role in ensuring optimal healing, sustained weight loss, and overall well-being. In this chapter, we will delve into the nuances of the gastric sleeve diet, from preparing for surgery with dietary guidelines to navigating the various post-surgery dietary phases and understanding the specific nutritional requirements for gastric sleeve patients.

Preparing for Surgery: Dietary Guidelines

Before the actual surgical date, a period of preparation is essential to optimize the outcomes of gastric sleeve surgery. This preparation extends to dietary habits, with specific guidelines aimed at both physically and mentally preparing individuals for the transformative journey ahead.

Healthy Eating Patterns: Transitioning to healthier eating habits before surgery sets the stage for post-surgery success. Emphasize a balanced diet rich in fruits, vegetables, lean proteins, and whole grains.

This not only aids in weight loss before surgery but also fosters a positive relationship with nutritious foods.

Hydration: Staying well-hydrated is crucial. Adequate water intake supports overall health and aids in flushing toxins from the body. Developing the habit of mindful hydration prepares individuals for the post-surgery emphasis on maintaining proper fluid levels.

Protein Intake: Protein is a cornerstone of pre-surgery preparation. Incorporating lean protein sources like poultry, fish, beans, and tofu helps preserve muscle mass and supports the body's healing processes. Protein-rich diets also contribute to a feeling of fullness, aiding in pre-surgery weight loss.

Vitamin and Mineral Supplementation: Depending on individual needs and pre-surgery nutritional assessments, healthcare providers may recommend vitamin and mineral supplements. Ensuring optimal levels of essential nutrients pre-surgery sets a foundation for a smoother recovery.

Mindful Eating Practices: Cultivating mindful eating habits involves savoring each bite, recognizing hunger and satiety cues, and avoiding emotional eating.

These practices contribute to a healthier relationship with food, which is invaluable throughout the gastric sleeve surgery journey.

Post-Surgery Dietary Phases

The post-surgery dietary phases are a gradual progression, allowing the body to adapt to its newly reduced stomach size and promoting healing. Each phase introduces specific food textures and consistencies, gradually reintroducing solid foods as the body adjusts. While individual timelines may vary, the general progression includes the following phases:

Clear Liquid Phase: Immediately after surgery, the initial phase involves clear liquids such as water, broth, and sugar-free gelatin. This phase helps prevent dehydration, provides essential hydration, and allows the stomach to heal.

Full Liquid Phase: Progressing from clear liquids, this phase includes protein shakes, low-fat milk, and strained soups. The emphasis remains on hydration and obtaining essential nutrients in a easily digestible form.

Pureed Food Phase: Gradually transitioning to a more diverse diet, this phase introduces pureed foods such as mashed vegetables, blended soups, and finely pureed proteins. The goal is to provide nutritional variety while maintaining a texture that is gentle on the healing stomach.

Soft Food Phase: This phase introduces soft, easily chewable foods like cooked vegetables, ground meats, and soft fruits. The emphasis is on ensuring that foods are thoroughly chewed to facilitate digestion.

Transition to Solid Foods: As the stomach continues to heal and adapt, solid foods are reintroduced. This phase involves incorporating a wider range of textures and consistencies, including lean proteins, whole grains, and a variety of fruits and vegetables.

Throughout these phases, it is crucial for individuals to follow their healthcare provider's guidance, attend regular check-ups, and listen to their bodies. Each phase serves as a building block, preparing the digestive system for the long-term changes associated with the gastric sleeve diet.

Nutritional Requirements for Gastric Sleeve Patients

Understanding the specific nutritional requirements for gastric sleeve patients is essential for long-term success and well-being. The surgery itself alters the digestive system, impacting the body's ability to absorb certain nutrients. Therefore, a balanced and nutrient-dense diet becomes paramount to prevent deficiencies and promote optimal health.

Protein: Protein is a cornerstone of the gastric sleeve diet. Adequate protein intake supports muscle preservation, aids in healing, and contributes to a feeling of fullness. Lean sources such as poultry, fish, tofu, and legumes are essential components of post-surgery meals.

Hydration: Maintaining proper hydration is crucial post-surgery. The reduced stomach size means that adequate fluid intake is vital for overall health. Sipping water throughout the day, avoiding sugary beverages, and prioritizing hydration support the body's various functions.

Vitamins and Minerals: Due to the altered digestive system, gastric sleeve patients may be at risk of vitamin and mineral deficiencies. Common supplements include vitamin B12, iron, calcium, and vitamin D. Regular monitoring of nutrient levels and adherence to supplementation recommendations are essential components of post-surgery care.

Fiber: Including fiber-rich foods in the diet supports digestive health and helps prevent constipation, a common concern post-surgery. Gradually introducing fiber from sources like fruits, vegetables, and whole grains ensures a well-balanced diet.

Portion Control and Mindful Eating: The reduced stomach size necessitates a shift towards smaller, more frequent meals. Practicing portion control and adopting mindful eating habits, such as eating slowly and savoring each bite, contribute to improved digestion and overall well-being.

Balanced Nutrition: Striking a balance between macronutrients (carbohydrates, proteins, and fats) is crucial.

The emphasis is on nutrient-dense, whole foods that provide essential vitamins and minerals without excessive calories. Incorporating a variety of colors and textures into meals ensures a diverse and enjoyable eating experience.

The gastric sleeve diet is not just a set of dietary guidelines but a transformative journey towards health and well-being. Embracing the process with a positive mindset, celebrating achievements, and focusing on nourishment can turn the dietary aspect of gastric sleeve surgery into a foundation for lasting health and vitality. As you navigate the various phases and nutritional requirements, remember that each step is a powerful investment in your long-term wellness, and the benefits extend far beyond the initial stages of the post-surgery period.

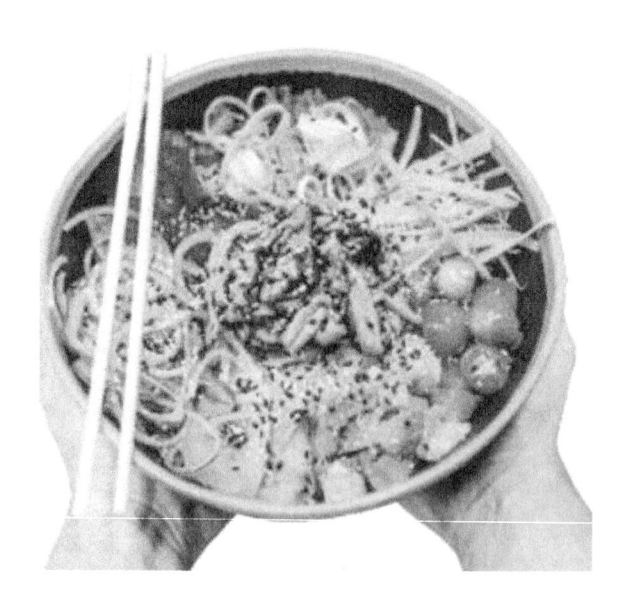

ESSENTIAL KITCHEN TOOLS AND INGREDIENTS

In the realm of post-gastric sleeve surgery nutrition, the kitchen becomes a sanctuary where healthy and flavorful meals take center stage. Equipping your kitchen with the right tools and stocking it with essential ingredients are pivotal steps towards making your culinary journey not only efficient but also enjoyable. In this chapter, we'll explore the must-have kitchen equipment, delve into the key ingredients for a bariatric-friendly pantry, and provide practical shopping tips to ensure you're well-prepared to create nourishing and delicious meals.

Must-Have Kitchen Equipment:

Blender or Food Processor: A high-quality blender or food processor is an invaluable asset in the post-gastric sleeve kitchen. It aids in creating smooth purees and blending ingredients for soups, smoothies, and other nutritious concoctions.

Digital Kitchen Scale: Precision in portion control is a cornerstone of post-surgery nutrition. A digital kitchen scale helps measure ingredients accurately, ensuring you stay within your recommended portion sizes.

Sharp Knives: Investing in a set of sharp knives makes food preparation more efficient and safer. From slicing vegetables to trimming lean proteins, a good set of knives is essential for creating well-prepared meals.

Non-Stick Cookware: Non-stick pans and pots facilitate cooking with minimal oil, making it easier to create healthy and delicious meals. They are especially useful when cooking lean proteins or sautéing vegetables.

Steamer Basket: Steaming is a cooking method that preserves the nutritional content of foods. A steamer basket is excellent for preparing vegetables, lean proteins, and even grains, ensuring they retain their natural flavors and nutrients.

Measuring Cups and Spoons: Accurate measurements are crucial, particularly in the early phases of the post-surgery diet. Measuring cups and spoons help control portion sizes and maintain the nutritional balance of your meals.

Slow Cooker or Instant Pot: These kitchen wonders simplify meal preparation. Slow cookers and Instant Pots are ideal for creating flavorful, one-pot meals with minimal effort. They're particularly useful for busy days when you want a nutritious meal without extensive hands-on cooking.

Bariatric-Friendly Utensils: Consider utensils that make eating more comfortable post-surgery. Smaller-sized forks and spoons can help manage portion sizes, and utensils with ergonomic designs may enhance the dining experience.

Stocking Your Pantry with Healthy Ingredients:

Protein Sources:

- Lean meats such as chicken, turkey, and fish.
- Plant-based proteins like tofu, lentils, and beans.
- Protein powders or shakes for convenient protein supplementation.

Whole Grains and Complex Carbohydrates:

- Quinoa, brown rice, and whole-grain pasta.
- Rolled oats for a versatile and filling breakfast option.

- Whole-grain crackers or wraps for quick and healthy snacks.

Fruits and Vegetables:

- A variety of fresh or frozen fruits and vegetables to ensure a colorful and nutrient-rich diet.
- Leafy greens, berries, and citrus fruits for their antioxidant and vitamin content.
- Frozen vegetables for convenience and to minimize food waste.

Healthy Fats:

- Avocados for their creamy texture and heart-healthy monounsaturated fats.
- Nuts and seeds like almonds, chia seeds, and flaxseeds for added texture and nutritional value.
- Olive oil or avocado oil for cooking and dressing salads.

Dairy and Alternatives:

- Greek yogurt or low-fat yogurt for a protein-rich snack.
- Low-fat or plant-based milk for use in recipes or as a beverage.
- Cheese in moderation, choosing lower-fat varieties.

Herbs and Spices:

- Diverse herbs and spices to enhance the flavor of your meals without relying on excess salt or sugar.
- Essentials like garlic powder, cumin, paprika, and herbs like basil and thyme.

Low-Sugar Sauces and Condiments:

- Tomato sauce with no added sugar.
- Mustard, hot sauce, or vinegar for flavor without excess calories.
- Low-sodium soy sauce or tamari for a burst of umami.

Hydration Aids:

- Sugar-free or naturally flavored water enhancers to make hydration more enjoyable.
- Herbal teas for variety and hydration without added calories.

Shopping Tips for Bariatric-Friendly Foods:

Stick to the Perimeter: The perimeter of the grocery store typically houses fresh produce, lean proteins, and dairy. Focusing on these areas helps you make healthier choices and avoid highly processed foods.

Read Labels: Pay close attention to food labels, especially when selecting packaged items. Look for low-sugar, low-fat, and high-protein options. Be mindful of portion sizes and avoid products with excessive additives.

Prioritize Protein: When selecting meats, prioritize lean cuts and opt for skinless poultry. Consider plant-based protein sources like tofu and legumes for variety.

Embrace Frozen and Fresh Produce: Both frozen and fresh produce are excellent choices.

Frozen options can be more convenient and have a longer shelf life, while fresh produce provides a variety of textures and flavors.

Plan Ahead: Make a weekly meal plan before you go to the grocery shop. This helps create a focused shopping list and minimizes the chance of impulsive, less healthy choices.

Bulk Buying of Staples: Purchase staple items like grains, beans, and nuts in bulk. This can be cost-effective and ensures you always have the foundation for a nutritious meal at hand.

Opt for Whole Foods: whenever feasible, go for entire, unadulterated foods. These foods are rich in nutrients and contribute to a well-rounded and nourishing diet.

Stay Hydrated: Prioritize water and other low-calorie beverages over sugary drinks. Consider keeping a refillable water bottle with you to encourage consistent hydration.

Equipping your kitchen with essential tools and stocking it with nutritious ingredients sets the stage for success in your post-gastric sleeve journey.

With the right equipment and a well-stocked pantry, you'll find joy and creativity in preparing meals that not only meet your nutritional needs but also tantalize your taste buds. The combination of practical kitchen essentials and thoughtfully chosen ingredients will empower you to embrace a bariatric-friendly lifestyle with enthusiasm and confidence.

NUTRITIONAL GUIDANCE AND TIPS

Here, we delve into key aspects of nutritional guidance, emphasizing portion control, mindful eating, meeting micronutrient needs, and adapting the cookbook to individual dietary requirements.

Portion Control and Mindful Eating

One of the cornerstones of successful post-surgery nutrition is mastering portion control and embracing mindful eating. Gastric sleeve surgery reduces the stomach's capacity, making it crucial to savor every bite and make each one count. The recipes in this cookbook are thoughtfully crafted with appropriate portion sizes to align with the needs of gastric sleeve patients.

Understanding portion control isn't about restriction; it's about providing your body with the nutrients it requires while respecting its new limitations. By adopting mindful eating practices, you can cultivate a deeper connection with your food, fostering a sense of satisfaction and preventing overconsumption.

As you explore the delicious recipes within these pages, take the time to savor the flavors, appreciate the textures, and listen to your body's cues.

Tips for Portion Control:

Use Smaller Plates: Trick your mind into feeling satisfied with smaller portions by serving meals on smaller plates.

Chew Thoroughly: Slow down the eating process, allowing your body to recognize fullness signals.

Measure Ingredients: Be precise with recipe measurements to avoid unintentional overeating.

Hydrate: Drink water throughout meals to enhance feelings of fullness.

Meeting Micronutrient Needs

After gastric sleeve surgery, ensuring you meet your body's micronutrient needs becomes paramount. The reduction in stomach size may impact the absorption of certain vitamins and minerals. This cookbook is designed to incorporate ingredients rich in essential nutrients, aiding in a well-rounded and balanced post-surgery diet.

Key Micronutrients to Focus On:

Protein: Vital for muscle repair and overall body function, the recipes emphasize protein-packed ingredients such as lean meats, poultry, fish, tofu, and legumes.

Vitamins and Minerals: Incorporate a colorful array of fruits and vegetables to ensure a diverse range of vitamins and minerals, supporting your immune system and overall health.

Calcium and Vitamin D: Essential for bone health, recipes include dairy or fortified alternatives to meet these needs.

B Vitamins: Found in whole grains, lean meats, and leafy greens, these are crucial for energy metabolism.

Flexibility and Substitutions:

Vegetarian or Vegan Options: Many recipes provide alternatives for those following a plant-based lifestyle. Use plant-based proteins like tofu, tempeh, or lentils in place of meat.

Gluten-Free: For those with gluten sensitivities, explore the array of naturally gluten-free options and utilize gluten-free substitutes when necessary.

Low-Carb Modifications: Tailor recipes to lower carbohydrate intake by reducing or replacing certain ingredients. Emphasize non-starchy vegetables and lean proteins.

Allergen Considerations: Be mindful of allergens and adapt recipes accordingly. The cookbook offers guidance on common allergens and suggests suitable substitutes.

DELICIOUS AND POST-SURGERY RECIPES

BREAKFAST RECIPES

1. Berry Blast Protein Smoothie

Ingredients:

- A half-cup of frozen berry mixture (raspberries, blue berries, and strawberries)
- 1/2 cup Greek yogurt (non-fat or low-fat)
- One scoop of plan-based or whey protein powder.
- 1/2 cup almond milk (unsweetened)
- 1 tablespoon chia seeds (optional)

Preparation:

1. Blend all ingredients until smooth.
2. Add water or more almond milk to achieve your desired consistency.

Portion Size: 1 cup

Time: 5 minutes

Nutritional Information:

- Protein: 25g
- Carbohydrates: 20g
- Fat: 7g
- Fiber: 6g

2. Apple Cinnamon Protein Oatmeal

Ingredients:

- 1/4 cup old-fashioned oats
- 1/2 cup water or milk (unsweetened almond milk works well)
- 1/2 apple, diced
- 1 tablespoon protein powder
- 1/2 teaspoon cinnamon
- 1 teaspoon chia seeds

Preparation:

1. Cook oats in water or milk until soft.
2. Stir in diced apples, protein powder, cinnamon, and chia seeds.
3. Cook for an additional 2-3 minutes until apples are tender.

Portion Size: 1/2 cup

Time: 10 minutes

Nutritional Information:

- Protein: 15g
- Carbohydrates: 30g
- Fat: 5g
- Fiber: 6g

3. Spinach and Feta Egg Muffins

Ingredients:

- 2 large eggs
- 1/4 cup spinach, chopped
- 1 tablespoon feta cheese, crumbled
- Salt and pepper to taste

Preparation:

1. Preheat oven to 350°F (175°C).
2. In a bowl, whisk eggs and mix in chopped spinach, feta, salt, and pepper.
3. Pour mixture into muffin tin cups.
4. Bake the eggs for 15-20 minutes, or until they set.

Portion Size: 2 muffins

Time: 20 minutes

Nutritional Information:

- Protein: 18g
- Carbohydrates: 2g
- Fat: 12g
- Fiber: 1g

4. Chia Seed Pudding Parfait

Ingredients:

- 2 tablespoons chia seeds
- 1/2 cup unsweetened almond milk
- 1/4 cup Greek yogurt
- 1/2 cup mixed berries
- 1 tablespoon sliced almonds

Preparation:

1. Mix chia seeds and almond milk in a jar; refrigerate overnight.
2. In the morning, layer chia pudding with Greek yogurt, berries, and sliced almonds.

Portion Size: 1 cup

Time: Overnight (plus 5 minutes in the morning)

Nutritional Information:

- Protein: 12g
- Carbohydrates: 20g
- Fat: 10g
- Fiber: 10g

5. Cottage Cheese and Pineapple Protein Bowl

Ingredients:

- 1/2 cup low-fat cottage cheese
- 1/2 cup fresh pineapple chunks
- 1 tablespoon chopped walnuts
- Drizzle of honey (optional)

Preparation:

1. Mix cottage cheese and pineapple in a bowl.
2. Top with chopped walnuts and a drizzle of honey if desired.

Portion Size: 1 cup

Time: 5 minutes

Nutritional Information:

- Protein: 20g
- Carbohydrates: 25g
- Fat: 8g
- Fiber: 2g

6. Avocado and Turkey Breakfast Wrap

Ingredients:

- 1 small whole wheat or low-carb tortilla
- 2 slices turkey breast
- 1/4 avocado, sliced
- 1 egg, scrambled

Preparation:

1. Cook the scrambled egg.
2. Lay out the tortilla and add turkey, scrambled egg, and sliced avocado.
3. Roll into a wrap.

Portion Size: 1 wrap

Time: 10 minutes

Nutritional Information:

- Protein: 20g
- Carbohydrates: 20g
- Fat: 15g
- Fiber: 6g

7. Blueberry Protein Pancakes

Ingredients:

- 1/4 cup oat flour
- 1/4 cup cottage cheese
- 1/4 cup blueberries
- 1 egg
- 1/2 teaspoon baking powder

Preparation:

- Blend oat flour, cottage cheese, blueberries, egg, and baking powder until smooth.
- Pour onto a hot griddle to make small pancakes.

Portion Size: 2 pancakes

Time: 15 minutes

Nutritional Information:

- Protein: 15g
- Carbohydrates: 20g
- Fat: 7g
- Fiber: 3g

8. Greek Yogurt Parfait with Almond Granola

Ingredients:

- 1/2 cup Greek yogurt (non-fat)
- 1/4 cup almond granola
- 1/4 cup mixed berries
- 1 teaspoon honey

Preparation:

1. Layer Greek yogurt with almond granola and mixed berries.
2. Drizzle with honey before serving.

Portion Size: 1 cup

Time: 5 minutes

Nutritional Information:

- Protein: 18g
- Carbohydrates: 25g
- Fat: 6g
- Fiber: 4g

9. Quinoa Breakfast Bowl

Ingredients:

- 1/2 cup cooked quinoa
- 1/4 cup almond milk
- 1 tablespoon chopped nuts (almonds, walnuts)
- 1/2 banana, sliced
- Cinnamon for flavor

Preparation:

1. Combine cooked quinoa with almond milk.
2. Top with chopped nuts, sliced banana, and a sprinkle of cinnamon.

Portion Size: 1 cup

Time: 10 minutes

Nutritional Information:

- Protein: 10g
- Carbohydrates: 30g
- Fat: 8g
- Fiber: 4g

10. Savory Veggie and Cheese Omelette

Ingredients:

- 2 large eggs
- 1/4 cup diced bell peppers
- 1/4 cup diced tomatoes
- 1/4 cup shredded low-fat cheese
- Salt and pepper to taste

Preparation:

1. Whisk eggs and pour into a hot, non-stick skillet.
2. Add bell peppers, tomatoes, cheese, salt, and pepper.
3. Fold the omelet in half and cook until eggs are set.

Portion Size: 1 omelet

Time: 10 minutes

Nutritional Information:

- Protein: 20g
- Carbohydrates: 5g
- Fat: 12g
- Fiber: 2g

LUNCH RECIPES

1. Grilled Chicken Salad with Balsamic Vinaigrette

Ingredients:

- 4 oz grilled chicken breast, sliced
- 2 cups mixed salad greens
- 1/2 cup cherry tomatoes, halved
- 1/4 cup cucumber, sliced
- 1 tablespoon feta cheese, crumbled
- 1 tablespoon balsamic vinaigrette

Preparation:

1. Grill chicken breast until fully cooked.
2. Assemble salad with mixed greens, cherry tomatoes, cucumber, and grilled chicken.
3. Top with feta cheese and drizzle with balsamic vinaigrette.

Portion Size: 1.5 cups

Time: 20 minutes

Nutritional Information:

- Protein: 30g
- Carbohydrates: 10g
- Fat: 8g
- Fiber: 3g

2. Quinoa and Black Bean Bowl

Ingredients:

- 1/2 cup cooked quinoa
- 1/2 cup black beans, drained and rinsed
- 1/4 cup corn kernels
- 1/4 cup diced bell peppers
- 1 tablespoon fresh cilantro, chopped
- 1 tablespoon lime juice

Preparation:

1. Cook quinoa according to package instructions.
2. In a bowl, mix cooked quinoa, black beans, corn, bell peppers, cilantro, and lime juice.

Portion Size: 1 cup

Time: 15 minutes

Nutritional Information:

- Protein: 15g
- Carbohydrates: 40g
- Fat: 2g
- Fiber: 8g

3. Salmon and Vegetable Stir-Fry

Ingredients:

- 4 oz salmon fillet, grilled or baked
- 1 cup broccoli florets
- 1/2 cup snap peas
- 1/4 cup carrots, julienned
- 1 tablespoon low-sodium soy sauce
- 1 teaspoon sesame oil

Preparation:

1. Grill or bake salmon until fully cooked.
2. In a wok or skillet, stir-fry broccoli, snap peas, and carrots in sesame oil.
3. Add cooked salmon and soy sauce, tossing until heated through.

Portion Size: 1.5 cups

Time: 25 minutes

Nutritional Information:

- Protein: 25g
- Carbohydrates: 15g
- Fat: 10g
- Fiber: 5g

4. Turkey and Veggie Lettuce Wraps

Ingredients:

- 4 oz ground turkey, cooked
- 1/2 cup bell peppers, diced
- 1/4 cup red onion, finely chopped
- 1/4 cup salsa
- 1 tablespoon Greek yogurt
- Lettuce leaves for wrapping

Preparation:

1. Cook ground turkey until browned.
2. Mix cooked turkey with bell peppers, red onion, salsa, and Greek yogurt.
3. Spoon the mixture into lettuce leaves, creating wraps.

Portion Size: 2 wraps

Time: 20 minutes

Nutritional Information:

- Protein: 20g
- Carbohydrates: 10g
- Fat: 8g
- Fiber: 3g

5. Vegetarian Quiche Cups

Ingredients:

- 2 large eggs
- 1/4 cup cottage cheese
- 1/4 cup spinach, chopped
- 1/4 cup cherry tomatoes, diced
- 1 tablespoon feta cheese, crumbled

Preparation:

1. Preheat oven to 350°F (175°C).
2. In a bowl, whisk eggs and mix in cottage cheese, spinach, tomatoes, and feta.
3. Pour the mixture into muffin tin cups.
4. Bake the eggs for 15 to 20 minutes, or until they set.

Portion Size: 2 quiche cups

Time: 25 minutes

Nutritional Information:

- Protein: 15g
- Carbohydrates: 5g
- Fat: 10g
- Fiber: 2g

6. Mediterranean Chickpea Salad

Ingredients:

- 1/2 cup canned chickpeas, drained and rinsed
- 1/4 cup cucumber, diced
- 1/4 cup cherry tomatoes, halved
- 2 tablespoons Kalamata olives, sliced
- 1 tablespoon feta cheese, crumbled
- 1 tablespoon olive oil
- 1 tablespoon lemon juice
- Fresh herbs (parsley, mint) for garnish

Preparation:

1. Combine chickpeas, cucumber, tomatoes, olives, and feta in a bowl.
2. Drizzle with olive oil and lemon juice.
3. Garnish with fresh herbs before serving.

Portion Size: 1 cup

Time: 15 minutes

Nutritional Information:

- Protein: 12g
- Carbohydrates: 20g
- Fat: 10g
- Fiber: 6g

7. Egg Salad Lettuce Wraps

Ingredients:

- 2 hard-boiled eggs, chopped
- 1 tablespoon Greek yogurt
- 1/4 cup celery, finely diced
- 1 tablespoon green onions, chopped
- Lettuce leaves for wrapping

Preparation:

1. In a bowl, mix chopped eggs, Greek yogurt, celery, and green onions.
2. Spoon the mixture into lettuce leaves, creating wraps.

Portion Size: 2 wraps

Time: 15 minutes

Nutritional Information:

- Protein: 15g
- Carbohydrates: 5g
- Fat: 10g
- Fiber: 2g

8. Shrimp and Avocado Zoodle Bowl

Ingredients:

- 4 oz shrimp, cooked
- 1 medium zucchini, spiralized
- 1/4 cup cherry tomatoes, halved
- 1/4 avocado, sliced
- 1 tablespoon cilantro, chopped
- 1 tablespoon lime juice

Preparation:

1. Cook shrimp until pink and opaque.
2. Spiralize zucchini and arrange on a plate.
3. Top with cooked shrimp, cherry tomatoes, avocado slices, cilantro, and lime juice.

Portion Size: 1.5 cups

Time: 20 minutes

Nutritional Information:

- Protein: 25g
- Carbohydrates: 15g
- Fat: 10g
- Fiber: 5g

9. Stuffed Bell Peppers with Ground Chicken

Ingredients:

- Two bell peppers, cut in half and seeded.
- 4 oz ground chicken, cooked
- 1/4 cup quinoa, cooked
- 1/4 cup black beans, drained and rinsed
- 1/4 cup salsa
- 1/4 cup shredded low-fat cheese

Preparation:

1. Preheat oven to 375°F (190°C).
2. In a bowl, mix cooked ground chicken, quinoa, black beans, salsa, and half of the shredded cheese.
3. Place a filling inside each half of a bell pepper.
4. Top with the remaining shredded cheese.
5. Bake for 25-30 minutes or until peppers are tender.

Portion Size: 1 pepper (2 halves)

Time: 40 minutes

Nutritional Information:

- Protein: 25g
- Carbohydrates: 25g
- Fat: 8g
- Fiber: 6g

10. Tuna and Avocado Lettuce Wraps

Ingredients:

- One can (5 oz) of a drained tuna in water.
- 1 tablespoon red onion, finely chopped
- 1 tablespoon celery, finely diced
- Lettuce leaves for wrapping

Preparation:

1. In a bowl, mix tuna, mashed avocado, red onion, and celery.
2. Spoon the mixture into lettuce leaves, creating wraps.

Portion Size: 2 wraps

Time: 15 minutes

Nutritional Information:

- Protein: 20g
- Carbohydrates: 5g
- Fat: 10g
- Fiber: 2g

DINNER RECIPES

1. Baked Lemon Herb Chicken

Ingredients:

- Four-ounce, skinless and boneless chicken breast.
- 1 tablespoon olive oil
- 1 teaspoon lemon zest
- 1 tablespoon fresh lemon juice
- 1 teaspoon dried herbs (rosemary, thyme, oregano)
- Salt and pepper to taste

Preparation:

1. Preheat oven to 400°F (200°C).
2. Mix olive oil, lemon zest, lemon juice, dried herbs, salt, and pepper.
3. Coat chicken with the mixture and bake for 20-25 minutes or until cooked through.

Portion Size: 1 chicken breast

Time: 30 minutes

Nutritional Information:

Protein: 30g, Carbohydrates: 1g, Fat: 8g, Fiber: 0g

2. Cauliflower Fried Rice with Shrimp

Ingredients:

- 4 oz shrimp, peeled and deveined
- 1 cup cauliflower rice
- 1/4 cup carrots, finely diced
- 1/4 cup peas
- 1/4 cup green onions, chopped
- 1 tablespoon low-sodium soy sauce
- 1 teaspoon sesame oil

Preparation:

1. Cook shrimp until pink and opaque.
2. In a skillet, stir-fry cauliflower rice, carrots, peas, and green onions in sesame oil.
3. Add cooked shrimp and soy sauce, tossing until heated through.

Portion Size: 1.5 cups

Time: 25 minutes

Nutritional Information:

- Protein: 25g
- Carbohydrates: 15g
- Fat: 8g
- Fiber: 5g

3. Turkey and Vegetable Skewers

Ingredients:

- 4 oz ground turkey, seasoned with herbs
- 1/2 bell pepper, cut into chunks
- 1/2 zucchini, sliced
- Cherry tomatoes
- 1 tablespoon olive oil
- 1 teaspoon Italian seasoning

Preparation:

1. Preheat grill or grill pan.
2. Form ground turkey into small skewers alternating with bell pepper, zucchini, and cherry tomatoes.
3. Grill skewers until turkey is fully cooked and vegetables are tender.

Portion Size: 2 skewers

Time: 20 minutes

Nutritional Information:

- Protein: 20g
- Carbohydrates: 10g
- Fat: 8g
- Fiber: 3g

4. Salmon and Asparagus Foil Packets

Ingredients:

- 4 oz salmon fillet
- Asparagus spears
- 1 tablespoon olive oil
- Lemon slices
- Fresh dill
- Salt and pepper to taste

Preparation:

1. Preheat oven to 400°F (200°C).
2. Place salmon on a piece of foil; add asparagus.
3. Drizzle with olive oil, add lemon slices, fresh dill, salt, and pepper.
4. Seal foil into packets and bake for 20 minutes.

Portion Size: 1 packet

Time: 25 minutes

Nutritional Information:

- Protein: 25g
- Carbohydrates: 5g
- Fat: 12g
- Fiber: 3g

5. Eggplant Lasagna with Ground Chicken

Ingredients:

- 1 medium eggplant, sliced
- 4 oz ground chicken, cooked
- 1 cup marinara sauce (low sugar)
- 1 cup part-skim ricotta cheese
- 1/2 cup mozzarella cheese, shredded
- Fresh basil for garnish

Preparation:

1. Preheat oven to 375°F (190°C).
2. Roast eggplant slices until tender.
3. In a baking dish, layer eggplant, ground chicken, marinara sauce, and ricotta.
4. Repeat layers, ending with a sprinkle of mozzarella.
5. Bake for 30 minutes or until bubbly and golden.

Portion Size: 1 cup

Time: 45 minutes

Nutritional Information:

- Protein: 20g
- Carbohydrates: 15g
- Fat: 10g
- Fiber: 5g

6. Chicken and Vegetable Stir-Fry

Ingredients:

- 4 oz chicken breast, thinly sliced
- 1 cup broccoli florets
- 1/2 cup snap peas
- 1/4 cup carrots, julienned
- 1/4 cup bell peppers, sliced
- 1 tablespoon low-sodium soy sauce
- 1 teaspoon sesame oil

Preparation:

1. Stir-fry chicken in sesame oil until browned.
2. Add broccoli, snap peas, carrots, and bell peppers.
3. Pour in soy sauce and stir until vegetables are tender.

Portion Size: 1.5 cups

Time: 20 minutes

Nutritional Information:

- Protein: 25g
- Carbohydrates: 10g
- Fat: 8g
- Fiber: 3g

7. Vegetarian Zucchini Noodles with Pesto

Ingredients:

- 1 medium zucchini, spiralized
- 2 tablespoons pesto sauce (homemade or store-bought)
- Cherry tomatoes, halved
- 1 tablespoon pine nuts
- Fresh basil for garnish

Preparation:

1. Spiralize zucchini and sauté in a pan until tender.
2. Toss with pesto sauce, cherry tomatoes, and pine nuts.
3. Garnish with fresh basil before serving.

Portion Size: 1.5 cups

Time: 15 minutes

Nutritional Information:

- Protein: 5g
- Carbohydrates: 10g
- Fat: 15g
- Fiber: 3g

8. Shredded Chicken Lettuce Wraps

Ingredients:

- 4 oz shredded chicken breast
- 1/4 cup water chestnuts, diced
- 1/4 cup mushrooms, chopped
- 2 tablespoons low-sodium soy sauce
- 1 tablespoon hoisin sauce
- Lettuce leaves for wrapping

Preparation:

1. In a skillet, cook shredded chicken with water chestnuts and mushrooms.
2. Stir in soy sauce and hoisin sauce.
3. Spoon the mixture into lettuce leaves, creating wraps.

Portion Size: 2 wraps

Time: 20 minutes

Nutritional Information:

- Protein: 20g
- Carbohydrates: 10g
- Fat: 8g
- Fiber: 2g

9. Cabbage and Turkey Casserole

Ingredients:

- 4 oz ground turkey, cooked
- 2 cups cabbage, shredded
- 1/2 cup tomato sauce (low sugar)
- 1 teaspoon Italian seasoning
- 1/4 cup Parmesan cheese, grated

Preparation:

1. Preheat oven to 375°F (190°C).
2. In a baking dish, layer shredded cabbage, cooked ground turkey, tomato sauce, and Italian seasoning.
3. Top with grated Parmesan cheese.
4. Bake for 25-30 minutes or until bubbly and golden.

Portion Size: 1 cup

Time: 40 minutes

Nutritional Information:

- Protein: 20g
- Carbohydrates: 10g
- Fat: 8g
- Fiber: 4g

10. Cilantro Lime Grilled Shrimp Salad

Ingredients:

- 4 oz shrimp, grilled
- 2 cups mixed salad greens
- 1/2 avocado, sliced
- 1/4 cup cherry tomatoes, halved
- 1/4 cup cucumber, sliced
- 1 tablespoon fresh cilantro, chopped
- 1 tablespoon lime juice
- 1 tablespoon olive oil

Preparation:

1. Grill shrimp until pink and opaque.
2. Assemble salad with mixed greens, avocado, cherry tomatoes, cucumber, and grilled shrimp.
3. Olive oil and lime juice should be drizzled on.

Portion Size: 1.5 cups

Time: 25 minutes

Nutritional Information:

Protein: 25g

Carbohydrates: 15g

Fat: 10g

Fiber: 5g

SNACK RECIPES

1. Greek Yogurt Parfait with Berries

Ingredients:

- 1/2 cup Greek yogurt (non-fat)
- 1/4 cup mixed berries (blueberries, strawberries, raspberries)
- 1 tablespoon almond granola
- 1 teaspoon honey (optional)

Preparation:

1. Arrange a mixture of berries on top of Greek yoghurt in a glass or bowl.
2. Top with almond granola and drizzle with honey if desired.

Portion Size: 1/2 cup

Time: 5 minutes

Nutritional Information:

- Protein: 15g
- Carbohydrates: 20g
- Fat: 5g
- Fiber: 4g

2. Cottage Cheese and Pineapple Bowl

Ingredients:

- 1/2 cup low-fat cottage cheese
- 1/2 cup fresh pineapple chunks
- 1 tablespoon sliced almonds
- Drizzle of honey (optional)

Preparation:

1. Combine cottage cheese and pineapple in a bowl.
2. Top with sliced almonds and a drizzle of honey if desired.

Portion Size: 1/2 cup

Time: 5 minutes

Nutritional Information:

- Protein: 15g
- Carbohydrates: 20g
- Fat: 5g
- Fiber: 2g

3. Hard-Boiled Egg and Avocado Slices

Ingredients:

- 2 hard-boiled eggs, sliced
- 1/4 avocado, sliced
- Salt and pepper to taste

Preparation:

1. Slice hard-boiled eggs and avocado.
2. Arrange on a plate and season with salt and pepper.

Portion Size: 1 egg and 1/4 avocado

Time: 10 minutes

Nutritional Information:

- Protein: 12g
- Carbohydrates: 5g
- Fat: 15g
- Fiber: 6g

4. Protein-Packed Trail Mix

Ingredients:

- 1/4 cup almonds
- 1/4 cup walnuts
- 2 tablespoons pumpkin seeds
- 2 tablespoons dark chocolate chips

Preparation:

1. Mix almonds, walnuts, pumpkin seeds, and dark chocolate chips in a bowl.
2. Portion into small snack-sized bags for easy grab-and-go.

Portion Size: 1/4 cup

Time: 5 minutes

Nutritional Information:

- Protein: 10g
- Carbohydrates: 10g
- Fat: 15g
- Fiber: 4g

5. Vegetable Sticks with Hummus

Ingredients:

- 1/2 cup baby carrots
- 1/2 cucumber, sliced
- 2 tablespoons hummus

Preparation:

1. Arrange baby carrots and cucumber slices on a plate.
2. Serve with hummus for dipping.

Portion Size: 1 cup vegetables and 2 tablespoons hummus

Time: 5 minutes

Nutritional Information:

- Protein: 5g
- Carbohydrates: 15g
- Fat: 8g
- Fiber: 6g

6. Turkey and Cheese Roll-Ups

Ingredients:

- 4 slices turkey breast
- 2 slices low-fat cheese
- 1 tablespoon mustard (optional)

Preparation:

1. Lay out turkey slices and place a cheese slice on each.
2. Roll up and secure with toothpicks.
3. Add mustard for extra flavor if desired.

Portion Size: 2 roll-ups

Time: 5 minutes

Nutritional Information:

- Protein: 15g
- Carbohydrates: 2g
- Fat: 8g
- Fiber: 0g

7. Caprese Skewers with Cherry Tomatoes and Mozzarella

Ingredients:

- Cherry tomatoes
- Fresh mozzarella balls
- Fresh basil leaves
- Balsamic glaze for drizzling

Preparation:

1. Thread cherry tomatoes, mozzarella balls, and fresh basil leaves onto small skewers.
2. Drizzle with balsamic glaze before serving.

Portion Size: 1 skewer

Time: 10 minutes

Nutritional Information:

- Protein: 5g
- Carbohydrates: 5g
- Fat: 8g
- Fiber: 1g

8. Edamame and Sea Salt

Ingredients:

- 1 cup edamame, steamed
- Sea salt to taste

Preparation:

1. Steam edamame according to package instructions.
2. Sprinkle with sea salt before serving.

Portion Size: 1 cup

Time: 10 minutes

Nutritional Information:

- Protein: 17g
- Carbohydrates: 15g
- Fat: 8g
- Fiber: 8g

9. Baked Kale Chips

Ingredients:

- 2 cups kale, torn into pieces
- 1 tablespoon olive oil
- 1/2 teaspoon garlic powder
- 1/2 teaspoon onion powder
- Pinch of salt

Preparation:

1. Preheat oven to 350°F (175°C).
2. Toss kale with olive oil, garlic powder, onion powder, and salt.
3. Spread on a baking sheet and bake for 10-15 minutes until crispy.

Portion Size: 1 cup

Time: 15 minutes

Nutritional Information:

- Protein: 5g
- Carbohydrates: 10g
- Fat: 8g
- Fiber: 3g

10. Protein-Packed Cottage Cheese Bowl

Ingredients:

- 1/2 cup low-fat cottage cheese
- 1/4 cup sliced strawberries
- 1 tablespoon chopped nuts (almonds, walnuts)
- Drizzle of honey (optional)

Preparation:

1. In a bowl, combine cottage cheese, sliced strawberries, and chopped nuts.
2. Drizzle with honey for sweetness if desired.

Portion Size: 1/2 cup

Time: 5 minutes

Nutritional Information:

- Protein: 15g
- Carbohydrates: 15g
- Fat: 8g
- Fiber: 2g

DESSERT AND TREAT RECIPES

1. Chia Seed Pudding with Berries

Ingredients:

- 2 tablespoons chia seeds
- 1/2 cup almond milk
- 1/4 teaspoon vanilla extract
- Mixed berries for topping

Preparation:

1. Mix chia seeds, almond milk, and vanilla extract in a bowl.
2. Refrigerate for at least 2 hours or overnight until it thickens.
3. Top with mixed berries before serving.

Portion Size: 1/2 cup

Time: 2 hours (including chilling time)

Nutritional Information:

- Protein: 5g
- Carbohydrates: 15g
- Fat: 8g
- Fiber: 8g

2. Baked Apple with Cinnamon

Ingredients:

- 1 medium apple, cored and sliced
- 1/2 teaspoon cinnamon
- 1 teaspoon lemon juice
- 1 tablespoon chopped nuts (walnuts or almonds)

Preparation:

1. Preheat oven to 375°F (190°C).
2. Toss apple slices with cinnamon and lemon juice.
3. Bake for 15-20 minutes until apples are tender.
4. Sprinkle with chopped nuts before serving.

Portion Size: 1/2 apple

Time: 20 minutes

Nutritional Information:

- Protein: 2g
- Carbohydrates: 20g
- Fat: 5g
- Fiber: 4g

3. Protein-Packed Chocolate Mousse

Ingredients:

- 1/2 cup Greek yogurt (non-fat)
- 1 tablespoon unsweetened cocoa powder
- 1 tablespoon honey
- 1/2 teaspoon vanilla extract

Preparation:

1. Mix Greek yogurt, cocoa powder, honey, and vanilla extract in a bowl.
2. Refrigerate for 1-2 hours until it reaches mousse-like consistency.

Portion Size: 1/2 cup

Time: 2 hours (including chilling time)

Nutritional Information:

- Protein: 15g
- Carbohydrates: 20g
- Fat: 5g
- Fiber: 2g

4. Frozen Banana Bites

Ingredients:

- 1 banana, sliced
- 2 tablespoons peanut butter
- Dark chocolate chips (optional)

Preparation:

1. Spread peanut butter on banana slices.
2. Sandwich slices together and freeze.
3. Optionally, dip frozen bites in melted dark chocolate.

Portion Size: 1 banana (sliced)

Time: 2 hours (including freezing time)

Nutritional Information:

- Protein: 5g
- Carbohydrates: 25g
- Fat: 10g
- Fiber: 4g

5. Coconut and Almond Energy Balls

Ingredients:

- 1/2 cup almonds, finely chopped
- 1/4 cup unsweetened shredded coconut
- 2 tablespoons almond butter
- 1 tablespoon honey
- 1/4 teaspoon vanilla extract

Preparation:

1. Combine chopped almonds, shredded coconut, almond butter, honey, and vanilla extract in a bowl.
2. Form into small balls and refrigerate for 1 hour.

Portion Size: 2 energy balls

Time: 1 hour (including chilling time)

Nutritional Information:

- Protein: 7g
- Carbohydrates: 10g
- Fat: 10g
- Fiber: 3g

6. Yogurt and Berry Parfait

Ingredients:

- 1/2 cup Greek yogurt (non-fat)
- 1/4 cup mixed berries (blueberries, strawberries)
- 1 tablespoon granola (low sugar)

Preparation:

1. Arrange a mixture of berries on top of Greek yoghourt in a glass or bowl.
2. Top with a sprinkle of granola.

Portion Size: 1/2 cup

Time: 5 minutes

Nutritional Information:

- Protein: 10g
- Carbohydrates: 15g
- Fat: 3g
- Fiber: 2g

7. Pumpkin Spice Protein Bites

Ingredients:

- 1/2 cup canned pumpkin puree
- 1/4 cup protein powder (vanilla or pumpkin spice)
- 2 tablespoons almond flour
- 1 tablespoon maple syrup
- 1/2 teaspoon pumpkin pie spice

Preparation:

1. Mix pumpkin puree, protein powder, almond flour, maple syrup, and pumpkin pie spice in a bowl.
2. Form into small bites and refrigerate for 1 hour.

Portion Size: 2 bites

Time: 1 hour (including chilling time)

Nutritional Information:

- Protein: 10g
- Carbohydrates: 10g
- Fat: 4g
- Fiber: 2g

8. Avocado Chocolate Mousse

Ingredients:

- 1 ripe avocado
- 2 tablespoons unsweetened cocoa powder
- 2 tablespoons maple syrup
- 1/2 teaspoon vanilla extract

Preparation:

1. Blend avocado, cocoa powder, maple syrup, and vanilla extract until smooth.
2. Refrigerate for 1-2 hours before serving.

Portion Size: 1/2 cup

Time: 2 hours (including chilling time)

Nutritional Information:

- Protein: 3g
- Carbohydrates: 20g
- Fat: 10g
- Fiber: 6g

9. Berry Sorbet

Ingredients:

- 1 cup mixed berries (frozen)
- 1 tablespoon lemon juice
- 1-2 tablespoons honey

Preparation:

1. Blend frozen berries, lemon juice, and honey until smooth.
2. Freeze for 2 hours, stirring every 30 minutes.

Portion Size: 1/2 cup

Time: 2.5 hours (including freezing time)

Nutritional Information:

- Protein: 2g
- Carbohydrates: 20g
- Fat: 0g
- Fiber: 4g

10. Almond Butter Stuffed Dates

Ingredients:

- 4 Medjool dates, pitted
- 2 tablespoons almond butter
- Sea salt for sprinkling

Preparation:

1. Cut dates in half and fill each with a teaspoon of almond butter.
2. Add a small amount of sea salt on top.

Portion Size: 4 stuffed dates

Time: 10 minutes

Nutritional Information:

- Protein: 5g
- Carbohydrates: 30g
- Fat: 10g
- Fiber: 4g

BARIATRIC-FRIENDLY SOUPS AND SALADS

1. Tomato Basil Soup

Ingredients:

- 1 cup fresh tomatoes, diced
- 1/2 cup low-sodium vegetable broth
- 1/4 cup fresh basil, chopped
- 1 clove garlic, minced
- Salt and pepper to taste

Preparation:

1. In a saucepan, combine tomatoes, vegetable broth, basil, and garlic.
2. Simmer for 15-20 minutes until tomatoes are tender.
3. After blending until smooth, add salt and pepper to taste.

Portion Size: 1 cup

Time: 25 minutes

Nutritional Information:

- Protein: 2g
- Carbohydrates: 10g
- Fat: 1g
- Fiber: 3g

2. Chicken and Vegetable Soup

Ingredients:

- 4 oz cooked chicken breast, shredded
- 1 cup mixed vegetables (carrots, celery, zucchini)
- 4 cups low-sodium chicken broth
- 1 teaspoon dried thyme
- Salt and pepper to taste

Preparation:

1. In a pot, combine shredded chicken, mixed vegetables, chicken broth, thyme, salt, and pepper.
2. Simmer for 20-25 minutes until vegetables are tender.

Portion Size: 1 cup

Time: 30 minutes

Nutritional Information:

- Protein: 15g
- Carbohydrates: 10g
- Fat: 2g
- Fiber: 3g

3. Spinach and Feta Salad

Ingredients:

- 2 cups fresh spinach
- 1/4 cup crumbled feta cheese
- 1/4 cup cherry tomatoes, halved
- 2 tablespoons balsamic vinaigrette

Preparation:

1. Toss fresh spinach, feta cheese, and cherry tomatoes in a bowl.
2. Drizzle with balsamic vinaigrette before serving.

Portion Size: 1 cup

Time: 10 minutes

Nutritional Information:

- Protein: 5g
- Carbohydrates: 8g
- Fat: 7g
- Fiber: 3g

4. Broccoli Cheddar Soup

Ingredients:

- 1 cup broccoli florets
- 1/2 cup low-fat cheddar cheese, shredded
- 2 cups low-sodium vegetable broth
- 1/4 cup onion, diced
- 1 clove garlic, minced

Preparation:

1. In a pot, combine broccoli, cheddar cheese, vegetable broth, onion, and garlic.
2. Simmer for 15-20 minutes until broccoli is tender.

Portion Size: 1 cup

Time: 25 minutes

Nutritional Information:

- Protein: 10g
- Carbohydrates: 12g
- Fat: 5g
- Fiber: 4g

5. Turkey and Cranberry Salad

Ingredients:

- 4 oz roasted turkey breast, sliced
- 1/4 cup dried cranberries
- 2 cups mixed salad greens
- 2 tablespoons vinaigrette dressing

Preparation:

1. Arrange turkey slices, dried cranberries, and mixed salad greens on a plate.
2. Drizzle with vinaigrette dressing.

Portion Size: 1.5 cups

Time: 15 minutes

Nutritional Information:

- Protein: 20g
- Carbohydrates: 15g
- Fat: 8g
- Fiber: 4g

6. Cauliflower and Leek Soup

Ingredients:

- 2 cups cauliflower florets
- 1 leek, sliced
- 4 cups low-sodium vegetable broth
- 1/4 cup Greek yogurt (non-fat)
- Fresh chives for garnish

Preparation:

1. In a pot, combine cauliflower, leek, vegetable broth, and Greek yogurt.
2. Simmer for 20-25 minutes until cauliflower is soft.
3. Blend until smooth and garnish with fresh chives.

Portion Size: 1 cup

Time: 30 minutes

Nutritional Information:

- Protein: 5g
- Carbohydrates: 10g
- Fat: 1g
- Fiber: 4g

7. Shrimp and Avocado Salad

Ingredients:

- 4 oz grilled shrimp
- 1/2 avocado, sliced
- 2 cups mixed salad greens
- 1 tablespoon lime vinaigrette

Preparation:

1. Grill shrimp until pink and opaque.
2. Assemble salad with grilled shrimp, avocado slices, and mixed salad greens.
3. Drizzle with lime vinaigrette.

Portion Size: 1.5 cups

Time: 20 minutes

Nutritional Information:

- Protein: 25g
- Carbohydrates: 10g
- Fat: 15g
- Fiber: 5g

8. Butternut Squash Soup

Ingredients:

- 2 cups butternut squash, diced
- 1/2 cup onion, chopped
- 4 cups low-sodium vegetable broth
- 1/4 teaspoon nutmeg
- Salt and pepper to taste

Preparation:

1. In a pot, combine butternut squash, onion, vegetable broth, nutmeg, salt, and pepper.
2. Simmer for 25-30 minutes until squash is tender.
3. Blend until smooth.

Portion Size: 1 cup

Time: 35 minutes

Nutritional Information:

- Protein: 3g
- Carbohydrates: 15g
- Fat: 1g
- Fiber: 4g

9. Quinoa and Chickpea Salad

Ingredients:

- 1/2 cup cooked quinoa
- 1/2 cup canned chickpeas, drained and rinsed
- 1/4 cup cucumber, diced
- 1/4 cup cherry tomatoes, halved
- 2 tablespoons lemon-tahini dressing

Preparation:

1. In a bowl, combine cooked quinoa, chickpeas, cucumber, and cherry tomatoes.
2. Drizzle with lemon-tahini dressing.

Portion Size: 1 cup

Time: 15 minutes

Nutritional Information:

- Protein: 8g
- Carbohydrates: 25g
- Fat: 6g
- Fiber: 6g

10. Asparagus and Mushroom Soup

Ingredients:

- 1 cup asparagus, chopped
- 1 cup mushrooms, sliced
- 4 cups low-sodium vegetable broth
- 1/4 cup low-fat cream cheese
- Fresh parsley for garnish

Preparation:

1. In a pot, combine asparagus, mushrooms, vegetable broth, and cream cheese.
2. Simmer for 20-25 minutes until vegetables are tender.
3. Garnish with fresh parsley before serving.

Portion Size: 1 cup

Time: 30 minutes

Nutritional Information:

- Protein: 6g
- Carbohydrates: 10g
- Fat: 4g
- Fiber: 3g

30-DAY MEAL PLAN

DAY 1

BREAKFAST: Berry Blast Protein Smoothie

LUNCH: Tuna and Avocado Lettuce Wraps

DINNER: Baked Lemon Herb Chicken

SNACK: Protein-Packed Cottage Cheese Bow

DESSERT: Chia Seed Pudding with Berries

DAY 2

BREAKFAST: Apple Cinnamon Protein Oatmeal

LUNCH: Stuffed Bell Peppers with Ground Chicken

DINNER: Cauliflower Fried Rice with Shrimp

SNACK: Baked Kale Chips

DESSERT: Baked Apple with Cinnamon

DAY 3

BREAKFAST: Spinach and Feta Egg Muffins

LUNCH: Shrimp and Avocado Zoodle Bowl

DINNER: Turkey and Vegetable Skewers

SNACK: Edamame and Sea Salt

DESSERT: Protein-Packed Chocolate Mousse

DAY 4

BREAKFAST: Chia Seed Pudding Parfait

LUNCH: Egg Salad Lettuce Wraps

DINNER: Salmon and Asparagus Foil Packets

SNACK: Caprese Skewers with Cherry Tomatoes and Mozzarella

DESSERT: Frozen Banana Bites

DAY 5

BREAKFAST: Cottage Cheese and Pineapple Protein Bowl

LUNCH: Mediterranean Chickpea Salad

DINNER: Eggplant Lasagna with Ground Chicken

SNACK: Turkey and Cheese Roll-Ups

DESSERT: Coconut and Almond Energy Balls

DAY 6

BREAKFAST: Avocado and Turkey Breakfast Wrap

LUNCH: Vegetarian Quiche Cups

DINNER: Chicken and Vegetable Stir-Fry

SNACK: Vegetable Sticks with Hummus

DESSERT: Yogurt and Berry Parfait

DAY 7

BREAKFAST: Blueberry Protein Pancakes

LUNCH: Turkey and Veggie Lettuce Wraps

DINNER: Vegetarian Zucchini Noodles with Pesto

SNACK: Protein-Packed Trail Mix

DESSERT: Pumpkin Spice Protein Bites

DAY 8

BREAKFAST: Greek Yogurt Parfait with Almond Granola

LUNCH: Salmon and Vegetable Stir-Fry

DINNER: Shredded Chicken Lettuce Wraps

SNACK: Hard-Boiled Egg and Avocado Slices

DESSERT: Avocado Chocolate Mousse

DAY 9

BREAKFAST: Quinoa Breakfast Bowl

LUNCH: Quinoa and Black Bean Bowl

DINNER: Cabbage and Turkey Casserole

SNACK: Cottage Cheese and Pineapple Bowl

DESSERT: Berry Sorbet

DAY 10

BREAKFAST: Savory Veggie and Cheese Omelette

LUNCH: Grilled Chicken Salad with Balsamic Vinaigrette

DINNER: Cilantro Lime Grilled Shrimp Salad

SNACK: Greek Yogurt Parfait with Berries

DESSERT: Almond Butter Stuffed Dates

DAY 11

BREAKFAST: Berry Blast Protein Smoothie

LUNCH: Tuna and Avocado Lettuce Wraps

DINNER: Baked Lemon Herb Chicken

SNACK: Protein-Packed Cottage Cheese Bow

DESSERT: Chia Seed Pudding with Berries

DAY 12

BREAKFAST: Apple Cinnamon Protein Oatmeal

LUNCH: Stuffed Bell Peppers with Ground Chicken

DINNER: Cauliflower Fried Rice with Shrimp

SNACK: Baked Kale Chips

DESSERT: Baked Apple with Cinnamon

DAY 13

BREAKFAST: Spinach and Feta Egg Muffins

LUNCH: Asparagus and Mushroom Soup

DINNER: Turkey and Vegetable Skewers

SNACK: Edamame and Sea Salt

DESSERT: Protein-Packed Chocolate Mousse

DAY 14

BREAKFAST: Chia Seed Pudding Parfait

LUNCH: Egg Salad Lettuce Wraps

DINNER: Salmon and Asparagus Foil Packets

SNACK: Caprese Skewers with Cherry Tomatoes and Mozzarella

DESSERT: Frozen Banana Bites

DAY 15

BREAKFAST: Cottage Cheese and Pineapple Protein Bowl

LUNCH: Mediterranean Chickpea Salad

DINNER: Eggplant Lasagna with Ground Chicken

SNACK: Turkey and Cheese Roll-Ups

DESSERT: Coconut and Almond Energy Balls

DAY 16

BREAKFAST: Avocado and Turkey Breakfast Wrap

LUNCH: Tomato Basil Soup

DINNER: Chicken and Vegetable Stir-Fry

SNACK: Vegetable Sticks with Hummus

DESSERT: Yogurt and Berry Parfait

DAY 17

BREAKFAST: Blueberry Protein Pancakes

LUNCH: Turkey and Veggie Lettuce Wraps

DINNER: Chicken and Vegetable Soup

SNACK: Protein-Packed Trail Mix

DESSERT: Pumpkin Spice Protein Bites

DAY 18

BREAKFAST: Greek Yogurt Parfait with Almond Granola

LUNCH: Salmon and Vegetable Stir-Fry

DINNER: Shredded Chicken Lettuce Wraps

SNACK: Hard-Boiled Egg and Avocado Slices

DESSERT: Avocado Chocolate Mousse

DAY 19

BREAKFAST: Quinoa Breakfast Bowl

LUNCH: Spinach and Feta Salad

DINNER: Cabbage and Turkey Casserole

SNACK: Cottage Cheese and Pineapple Bowl

DESSERT: Berry Sorbet

DAY 20

BREAKFAST: Savory Veggie and Cheese Omelette

LUNCH: Grilled Chicken Salad with Balsamic Vinaigrette

DINNER: Cilantro Lime Grilled Shrimp Salad

SNACK: Greek Yogurt Parfait with Berries

DESSERT: Almond Butter Stuffed Dates

DAY 21

BREAKFAST: Berry Blast Protein Smoothie

LUNCH: Broccoli Cheddar Soup

DINNER: Baked Lemon Herb Chicken

SNACK: Protein-Packed Cottage Cheese Bow

DESSERT: Chia Seed Pudding with Berries

DAY 22

BREAKFAST: Apple Cinnamon Protein Oatmeal

LUNCH: Stuffed Bell Peppers with Ground Chicken

DINNER: Cauliflower Fried Rice with Shrimp

SNACK: Baked Kale Chips

DESSERT: Baked Apple with Cinnamon

DAY 23

BREAKFAST: Spinach and Feta Egg Muffins

LUNCH: Shrimp and Avocado Zoodle Bowl

DINNER: Turkey and Cranberry Salad

SNACK: Edamame and Sea Salt

DESSERT: Protein-Packed Chocolate Mousse

DAY 24

BREAKFAST: Chia Seed Pudding Parfait

LUNCH: Egg Salad Lettuce Wraps

DINNER: Cauliflower and Leek Soup

SNACK: Caprese Skewers with Cherry Tomatoes and Mozzarella

DESSERT: Frozen Banana Bites

DAY 25

BREAKFAST: Cottage Cheese and Pineapple Protein Bowl

LUNCH: Mediterranean Chickpea Salad

DINNER: Eggplant Lasagna with Ground Chicken

SNACK: Turkey and Cheese Roll-Ups

DESSERT: Coconut and Almond Energy Balls

DAY 26

BREAKFAST: Avocado and Turkey Breakfast Wrap

LUNCH: Vegetarian Quiche Cups

DINNER: Chicken and Vegetable Stir-Fry

SNACK: Vegetable Sticks with Hummus

DESSERT: Yogurt and Berry Parfait

DAY 27

BREAKFAST: Blueberry Protein Pancakes

LUNCH: Shrimp and Avocado Salad

DINNER: Vegetarian Zucchini Noodles with Pesto

SNACK: Protein-Packed Trail Mix

DESSERT: Pumpkin Spice Protein Bites

DAY 28

BREAKFAST: Greek Yogurt Parfait with Almond Granola

LUNCH: Salmon and Vegetable Stir-Fry

DINNER: Shredded Chicken Lettuce Wraps

SNACK: Hard-Boiled Egg and Avocado Slices

DESSERT: Avocado Chocolate Mousse

DAY 29

BREAKFAST: Quinoa Breakfast Bowl

LUNCH: Butternut Squash Soup

DINNER: Cabbage and Turkey Casserole

SNACK: Cottage Cheese and Pineapple Bowl

DESSERT: Berry Sorbet

DAY 30

BREAKFAST: Savory Veggie and Cheese Omelette

LUNCH: Quinoa and Chickpea Salad

DINNER: Cilantro Lime Grilled Shrimp Salad

SNACK: Greek Yogurt Parfait with Berries

DESSERT: Almond Butter Stuffed Dates

CONCLUSION

This Gastric Sleeve Bariatric Cookbook is not merely a compilation of recipes but a holistic guide crafted with your well-being in mind. As you embark on this post-surgery journey, consider this cookbook as your faithful companion, offering not only nourishing and delicious recipes but also invaluable insights into portion control, mindful eating, and meeting your micronutrient needs.

Through these pages, we invite you to savor the flavors, embrace the joy of mindful cooking, and relish the transformation that each recipe brings. The culinary adventure within these covers is not just about fueling your body; it's a celebration of your commitment to health and self-care.

Remember, this journey is uniquely yours. The adaptability of these recipes allows for personalization, ensuring that your dietary preferences and requirements are seamlessly integrated into your daily meals.

As you navigate through the recipes, let the vibrant colors, rich textures, and enticing aromas inspire you. This cookbook is more than a manual; it's an invitation to explore, create, and savor the transformative power of wholesome, bariatric-friendly meals.

In the spirit of embracing this new chapter, relish the process of discovering foods that not only support rapid weight loss but also contribute to your overall well-being. Let each meal be a mindful celebration, a step towards reclaiming health, and an opportunity to foster a positive relationship with food.

We extend our warmest wishes for a successful and fulfilling journey. May the recipes within these pages bring you joy, nourishment, and a renewed sense of vitality. Here's to your health, happiness, and the delicious adventure that lies ahead.

Happy cooking, and may each bite be a celebration of your commitment to a healthier and happier you!

WEEKLY MEAL PLANNER

WEEKLY MEAL JOURNAL

WEEK _____   MONTH _____

MONDAY

TUESDAY

WEDNESDAY

THURSDAY

FRIDAY

SATURDAY

SUNDAY

SHOPPING LIST
-
-
-
-
-
-
-
-

NOTES:

WEEKLY MEAL JOURNAL

WEEK _____ MONTH _____

MONDAY

TUESDAY

WEDNESDAY

THURSDAY

FRIDAY

SATURDAY

SUNDAY

SHOPPING LIST
-
-
-
-
-
-
-
-
-

NOTES:
-
-
-
-

WEEKLY MEAL JOURNAL

WEEK _____   MONTH _____

MONDAY

TUESDAY

WEDNESDAY

THURSDAY

FRIDAY

SATURDAY

SUNDAY

SHOPPING LIST
- ○ _____
- ○ _____
- ○ _____
- ○ _____
- ○ _____
- ○ _____
- ○ _____
- ○ _____

NOTES
- ○ _____
- ○ _____
- ○ _____
- ○ _____

WEEKLY MEAL JOURNAL

WEEK _____   MONTH _____

MONDAY

TUESDAY

WEDNESDAY

THURSDAY

FRIDAY

SATURDAY

SUNDAY

SHOPPING LIST
- _____
- _____
- _____
- _____
- _____
- _____
- _____
- _____

NOTES:
- _____
- _____
- _____
- _____

WEEKLY MEAL JOURNAL

WEEK _____ MONTH _____

MONDAY

TUESDAY

WEDNESDAY

THURSDAY

FRIDAY

SATURDAY

SUNDAY

SHOPPING LIST
-
-
-
-
-
-
-
-

NOTES
-
-
-
-

WEEKLY MEAL JOURNAL

WEEK ——————— MONTH ———————

MONDAY

TUESDAY

WEDNESDAY

THURSDAY

FRIDAY

SATURDAY

SUNDAY

SHOPPING LIST
- ○ _____
- ○ _____
- ○ _____
- ○ _____
- ○ _____
- ○ _____
- ○ _____
- ○ _____

NOTES:
- ○ _____
- ○ _____
- ○ _____
- ○ _____

WEEKLY MEAL JOURNAL

WEEK _____   MONTH _____

MONDAY

TUESDAY

WEDNESDAY

THURSDAY

FRIDAY

SATURDAY

SUNDAY

SHOPPING LIST
- _____
- _____
- _____
- _____
- _____
- _____
- _____
- _____

NOTES:
- _____
- _____
- _____
- _____

WEEKLY MEAL JOURNAL

WEEK _____   MONTH _____

MONDAY

TUESDAY

WEDNESDAY

THURSDAY

FRIDAY

SATURDAY

SUNDAY

SHOPPING LIST
- _____
- _____
- _____
- _____
- _____
- _____
- _____
- _____

NOTES:
- _____
- _____
- _____
- _____

WEEKLY MEAL JOURNAL

WEEK _____   MONTH _____

MONDAY

TUESDAY

WEDNESDAY

THURSDAY

FRIDAY

SATURDAY

SUNDAY

SHOPPING LIST
-
-
-
-
-
-
-
-

NOTES
-
-
-
-

WEEKLY MEAL JOURNAL

WEEK ——————— MONTH ———————

MONDAY

TUESDAY

WEDNESDAY

THURSDAY

FRIDAY

SATURDAY

SUNDAY

SHOPPING LIST
-
-
-
-
-
-
-
-

NOTES:
-
-
-
-

WEEKLY MEAL JOURNAL

WEEK _____   MONTH _____

MONDAY

TUESDAY

WEDNESDAY

THURSDAY

FRIDAY

SATURDAY

SUNDAY

SHOPPING LIST
-
-
-
-
-
-
-
-

NOTES
-
-
-
-

WEEKLY MEAL JOURNAL

WEEK _____   MONTH _____

MONDAY

SATURDAY

TUESDAY

SUNDAY

WEDNESDAY

SHOPPING LIST
- _____
- _____
- _____
- _____
- _____
- _____
- _____
- _____

THURSDAY

FRIDAY

NOTES:
- _____
- _____
- _____
- _____